Rui Mateus Marques

Gastric Adenocarcinoma: role of CT in preoperative T and N
staging

AF190954

Rui Mateus Marques

Gastric Adenocarcinoma: role of CT in preoperative T and N staging

LAP LAMBERT Academic Publishing

Imprint

Any brand names and product names mentioned in this book are subject to trademark, brand or patent protection and are trademarks or registered trademarks of their respective holders. The use of brand names, product names, common names, trade names, product descriptions etc. even without a particular marking in this work is in no way to be construed to mean that such names may be regarded as unrestricted in respect of trademark and brand protection legislation and could thus be used by anyone.

Cover image: www.ingimage.com

Publisher:
LAP LAMBERT Academic Publishing
is a trademark of
Dodo Books Indian Ocean Ltd. and OmniScriptum S.R.L publishing group

120 High Road, East Finchley, London, N2 9ED, United Kingdom
Str. Armeneasca 28/1, office 1, Chisinau MD-2012, Republic of Moldova, Europe
Managing Directors: Ieva Konstantinova, Victoria Ursu
info@omniscriptum.com

Printed at: see last page
ISBN: 978-3-659-53286-3

Zugl. / Approved by: Lisboa, Universidade Nova, FCM, Diss. 2013

Contents

Aknowledgments

This work is dedicated to all professionals and family that supported me in this task.

A special thank to:

-Drs. Ana Vergamota, Rute Neves, Sara Jorge and all others Master Degree candidates for helping me in the work of the mastership.

- Prof. Pedro Caetano and Profª Maria Emília Monteiro for their enthusiasm and resilience in the Clinical Research Mastership Program.

-Colleagues and Technicians of the Radiology Department of Hospital de São José for the collaboration and assistance in the evaluation of the patients.

-The Multidisciplinary Gastro-esophageal Diseases Group of Centro Hospitalar de Lisboa Central, specially to Prof. Caldeira Fradique and Dr. Mário Oliveira for the analysis of datasets of Surgery and Pathology Departments.

-To my wife Elisa and our children João, Rui and Inês for their continuous inspiration.

Acronyms

AGC   Advanced Gastric Cancer

AJCC   American Joint Commission on Cancer

CT   Computed Tomography

DGS   Direcção Geral de Saúde (General Health Organization)

EBV   Ebstein-Barr Virus

EGC   Early Gastric Cancer

EGJ   Esophagogastric Junction

EUS   Endoscopic Ultrasound

GA   Gastric Adenocarcinoma

GE   General Electric

HP   Helycobacter Pylori

HU   Hounsfield Units

IARC   International Agency for Research on Cancer

JRSGC   Japanese Research Society for Gastric Cancer Classification

LOP   Left Posterior Oblique

MDCT   Multi-detector Computed Tomography

MPR   Multi-planar reformations

MRI   Magnetic Resonance Imaging

NCCN   National Cancer Comprehensive Network

N   Nodal

PET-CT   Positron Emission Tomography-Computed Tomography

TNM	Tumor Nodes Metastasis
T	Tumoral
UGE	Upper Gastrointestinal Endoscopy
UICC	International Union against Cancer
USA	United Sates of America
WHO	World Health Organization

Figures and Tables

Figure1: Incidence and Mortality related to Gastric Adenocarcinoma in Europe.

Table 1: UICC – TNM Staging Classification for Carcinoma of the Stomach.

Figure 2: Lymph nodes station numbers according to the Japanese Classification of Gastric Cancer, 14th edition (JGCA). Legends: See Table 1.

Table 2: Regional lymph nodes.

Figure 3: Normal study in a patient with early gastric cancer.

Figure 4: Example of GA after neoadjuvant chemotherapy.

Table 3: T staging correlation between MDCT/CT and Surgery for Gastric Adenocarcinoma in sixty nine patients.

Table 4: N staging correlation between MDCT/CT and Surgery for Gastric Adenocarcinoma in sixty nine patients.

Table 5: Separate evaluation of T Staging Sensitivity and Specificity.

Table 6: Separate evaluation of N Staging Sensitivity and Specificity.

Table 7: List of patients with diagnostic N2 Staging and N2/N3A pathologic staging (N3A patients 1 to 14 and N2 patients 15 to 21).

Table 8: N Staging with surrogate factor T4 changing T4/N2 diagnosis to T4/N3A diagnosis.

Table 9: Accuracy, Sensitivity and Specificity of N Staging, without and with Surrogate factors T4 and Diffuse type of Lauren´s Classification.

Introduction

Gastric adenocarcinoma (GA) is a worldwide significant health issue despite its declining incidence in Western World and the United States (Pinheiro et al 2002). It represents the fourth commonest neoplasm worldwide (McLoughin et al 2004, Kamangar et al 2006), the second commonest cause of death related to neoplasy (Kesley et al, 2005, Parkin, 2004) and the third commonest cause of death of cancer in Portugal (Globocan 2008). Although it is foreseen a gradual decline in the next ten years for incidence of gastric cancer outside the cardia in the Western World (de Vries et al, 2007), we have witnessed an increased absolute incidence of lesions at cardia in some western countries, perhaps explained by an increased prevalence of obesity (Merry et al, 2007).

In Europe, GA represents the fifth and sixth death cause by neoplastic disease in males and females respectively (IARC, 2008). Portugal is in fourth place concerning the incidence (27,1/100.000 habitants) and the sixth place concerning the mortality rate (22,7/100.0000 habitants) (Globocan, 2008) (Figure 1).

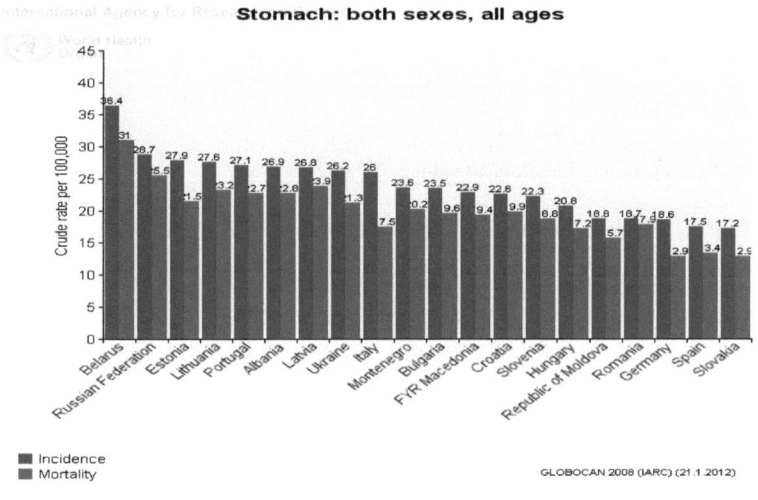

Figure 1: Incidence and Mortality related to Gastric Adenocarcinoma in Europe

7

Survival rate is related to the clinical stage after the diagnosis and curative surgery (including free margins resection and lymphadenectomy) with or without chemotherapy is considered the "gold standard" treatment method (Gore, 1997, Kim et al, 1999).

Even with a foreseeable trend in lowering of the mortality rate of GA in Portugal (Simões et al, 2008) with data supported by the D.G.S. (General Health Organization) of 24 by 100000 habitants in 1999, 17,5 by 100000 habitants in 2003 and forecast of 16,1 by 100000 habitants for 2015 (lower values compared with data from Globocan in 2008), GA mortality is higher than other common tumors. Such values demonstrate the biological aggressiveness of this entity that deserves a complementary research and work concerning the pathogeny, early diagnosis and treatment to ameliorate the patient prognosis.

The approach to the disease should consider patients evaluation by multidisciplinary teams for therapeutic decisions and there are international recommendations describing the diagnostic, staging and treatment criteria that should guide the orientation of patients suffering from GA (NCCN, 2010).

Epidemiology

A) Relationship to histological subtypes

The commonest classifications used for GA are the WHO (World Health Organization) and the Lauren´s Classification; this last one considers tumors of intestinal type, glandular developers, and diffuse type, composed by disorganized cells supported by cohesive and dense stroma, (Lauren, 1965). The intestinal type predominates in males, older ages, may be a follower of gastric atrophy or intestinal metaplasia and is more common in the highest incidence areas. Diffuse type is more common below 60 years of age, may be hereditary and its evolution is not preceded by intestinal metaplasia. Diffuse type predominates in low-risk areas and has became more frequent and with a more proximal distribution and tends to peritoneal dissemination while the intestinal type has became less frequent, more prone to environmental factors and favors the hematogeneous dissemination (Fenoglio et al, 2008).

8

The association of intestinal type to intestinal metaplasia may be susceptible to prediction through the evaluation of the malignant potential determined by biologic markers of genomic instability. As matter of a fact there are genetic modifications in intestinal metaplasia as p16 methylation (Dong et al, 2009) or reduced expression of e-cadherin in the mucosa of individuals infected with Helicobacter Pylori (Terres et al, 1998).

B) Relationship to the anatomic location of GA

The decreased incidence of GA, namely in the distal third, parallels the increased incidence of the tumor located in the cardia (Pera, 1993) and oesophageal adenocarcinoma (associated to obesity and reflux or Barrett´s esophagitis) in developed countries that occurred in the last 20 years. Cardia adenocarcinoma depicts the same epidemiological characteristics of distal esophageal adenocarcinoma and reflux esophagitis and many of the genetic and non genetical features suggest that carcinomas from the cardia and from extra-cardia location are different biological entities.

Etiopatogeny

The etiology of GA is considered multifactorial, depending on ambiental factors (high-sodium intake, benzopirens, endogenous and exogenous nitosamines tobacco, among others), infection by Helycobacter Pylori (HP), and genetic factors (patients with familiar history of cancer).

The Portuguese elevated incidence may be related to socio-economical and cultural factors. Nitrosamines have been considered for a long time carcinogenic agents of GA and they might be of endogenous or exogenous origin and the EPIC-EUROGAST study confirmed such relationship (Jacksyn et al, 2006). Salt-preserved foods and dietary nitrites incorporated in preserved meat are potentially carcinogenic and a diet with plenty of fruits and vegetables may significantly reduce the risk of gastric cancer (McCullough et al, 2001). The decreased incidence of GA may be explained by the widespread use of refrigerators, increasing intake of fresh fruit and vegetables and reducing intake of preserved meat. A case-control study performed in a Portuguese population demonstrated reduced incidence of gastric cancer in a population with elevated incidence of HP infection and a high intake of fruits and dairy products and low consumption of alcoholic beverages (Bastos et al, 2009).

HP infection represents an important risk factor with an increase of 2.8- to 6.0-fold (Sepulveda et al, 2011) and the risk is higher for women than men. HP gastritis may facilitate the growth of bacteria that catalyze the production of carcinogenic N-nitroso compounds (Sanduleanu et al, 2001). Tobacco smoking has been demonstrated as an important behavioral factor linked to GA (Ladeiras-Lopes et al, 2008). Ebstein-Barr Virus (VEB) is associated with tumors with lymphoid infiltration of the stroma, predominates in young male patients and has a better prognosis. Tumors related to VEB represent 10 % of total neoplasms but this percentage raise to 27-42% of tumors developing in postoperative stomach (Uozaki et al, 2008). There are mutations of cadherin-E in about 25% of families with a hereditary Autosomic Dominant variety of diffuse GA (Fitzgerald, 2004).

Prognostic factors

Despite recent diagnostic and therapeutic improvements, the prognosis of the disease is still grim, constituting the second commonest cause of death by neoplastic disease with a higher survival data in countries of high incidence compared to countries with low incidence (Verdechia et al, 2004). This fact may be explained by a higher incidence of lesions located in the antrum with a better prognosis, due to the implementation of large-scale population screening programs that underlies a diagnosis of lesions in early stage of development or adopting better surgical techniques performed by trained surgeons (Wang, 2010). Some factors related to the risk population may be responsible, as demonstrated with the higher survival rate of Americans of Asian origin compared to Americans of non-Asian origin (Theurer et al, 2000).

The most widely known and accepted prognostic factor for GA is the TNM classification even if it presents some limitations. The deepness of the tumor, its macroscopic appearance and size and its location were considered four independent correlation prognostic factors associated with the number of metastatic lymph nodes

(Shen et al, 1999). Several pathological factors have been associated with the prognosis like venous invasion (Preto et al, 2001), neural and lymphatic invasion, tumor length and its degree of differentiation. More recently, some oncobiologic markers have bee also used in the prognostic evaluation of the lesions (Pan et al, 2003, Nitti et al, 2008).

Staging

GC usually shows focal mural thickening with or without ulcerations, polypoid lesions, or diffuse mural thickening. The early gastric cancer (EGC) variant is defined as tumor confined to the mucosa or submucosa, regardless of the presence of lymph node metastasis, while the advanced gastric cancer form (AGC) invades the muscularis propria or the deeper wall layers (Katay, 2005, Ba-Ssalamah et al, 2003).

EGCs are classified into three types, as follows: type I, lesions are elevated and protrude >5 mm into the lumen; type IIa, lesions are elevated, but protrude less than 5 mm into the lumen; type IIb, lesions are essentially flat; type IIc, lesions are slightly depressed, but do not penetrate the muscularis mucosae; and type III lesions are true mucosal ulcers that penetrate the muscularis mucosae, but not the muscularis propria. AGCs can manifest as large, segmental, or diffuse wall thickening with or without ulceration or large, polypoid, and fungating lesions. Signet-ring cell cancer often manifests as obliteration of gastric folds and diffuse thickening of the gastric wall (linitis plastica).

Clinical staging has improved significantly with the complementary role of accessible and recent diagnostic modalities such as endoscopic ultrasound (EUS), multi--detector computed tomography (MDCT), combined positron emission tomography and computed tomography (PET-CT), magnetic resonance imaging (MRI) and laparoscopic imaging (Abdalla, 2004, Kwee, 2007, Weber, 2004)..

MDCT is currently an accessible and easy way to implement a T and N staging of the disease with an overall accuracy for T ranging from 42 to 83 % and accuracy, sensibility and specificity for N staging ranging respectively between 51 to 83,8%, 71,4 to 85,7% and 63,9 to 70% (D´Elia et al, 2000, Chen et al, 2007, Lee et al, 2012).

11

Clinical staging is important to determine the initial therapeutic strategy and two major classifications have been used. The Japanese Research Society for Gastric Cancer Classification (JRSGC, 1993) is based on the anatomical involvement of the neoplasm namely concerning its lymphatic dissemination and the classification accepted and sustained by the International Union for Cancer Control (UICC) and the AJCC (American Joint Committee on Cancer), the TNM system, with the latest revision presented in 2009 and 2010 (Sobin et al, 2009, Edge 2010) (Table 1)

PRIMARY TUMOR (T)	
❑ TX	Primary tumor cannot be assessed
❑ T0	No evidence of primary tumor
❑ Tis	Carcinoma *in situ*: intraepithelial tumor without invasion of the lamina propria
❑ T1	Tumor invades lamina propria, muscularis mucosae, or submucosa
❑ T1a	Tumor invades lamina propria or muscularis mucosae
❑ T1b	Tumor invades submucosa
❑ T2	Tumor invades muscularis propria
❑ T3	Tumor penetrates subserosal connective tissue without invasion of visceral peritoneum or adjacent structures[*],[**],[***]
❑ T4	Tumor invades serosa (visceral peritoneum) or adjacent structures[**],[***]
❑ T4a	Tumor invades serosa (visceral peritoneum)
❑ T4b	Tumor invades adjacent structures
	[*]A tumor may penetrate the muscularis propria with extension into the gastrocolic or gastrohepatic ligaments, or into the greater or lesser omentum, without perforation of the visceral peritoneum covering these structures. In this case, the tumor is classified T3. If there is perforation of the visceral peritoneum covering the gastric ligaments or the omentum, the tumor should be classified T4.
	[**]The adjacent structures of the stomach include the spleen, transverse colon, liver, diaphragm, pancreas, abdominal wall, adrenal gland, kidney, small intestine, and retroperitoneum.
	[***]Intramural extension to the duodenum or esophagus is classified by the depth of the greatest invasion in any of these sites, including the stomach.
REGIONAL LYMPH NODES (N)	
❑ NX	Regional lymph node(s) cannot be assessed
❑ N0	No regional lymph node metastasis[*]
❑ N1	Metastasis in 1 to 2 regional lymph nodes
❑ N2	Metastasis in 3 to 6 regional lymph nodes
❑ N3	Metastasis in 7 or more regional lymph nodes
❑ N3a	Metastasis in 7 to15 regional lymph nodes
❑ N3b	Metastasis in 16 or more regional lymph nodes
	[*] A designation of pN0 should be used if all examined lymph nodes are negative, regardless of the total number removed and examined.
DISTANT METASTASIS (M)	
❑ M0	No distant metastasis (no pathologic M0; use clinical M to complete stage group)
❑ M1	Distant metastasis

Table 1: UICC – TNM Staging Classification for Carcinoma of the Stomach (UICC, Seventh Edition, 2009)

In the Japanese Classification of Gastric Cancer by the Japanese Gastric Cancer Association (JGCA, 2010) lymph nodes surrounding stomach are divided into 20 groups and these are classified into three stations depending upon the location of the primary tumor (Figure 1, Table 2). This grouping system is based on the results of studies of lymphatic flow at various tumor sites, together with the observed survival associated with metastasis to each nodal station.

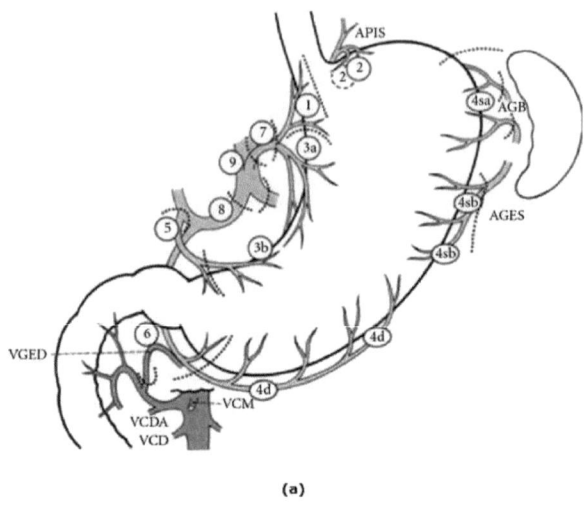

(a)

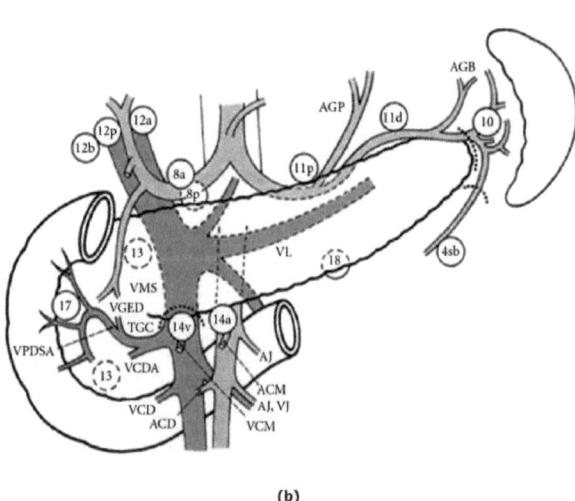

(b)

Figure 2: Lymph nodes group numbers according to the Japanese Classification of Gastric Cancer, 14th edition (JGCA). Legends: see Table 1.

No. 1	Right paracardial LN
No. 2	Lest paracardial LN
No. 3a	LN along the left gastric vessels
No. 3b	LN along the right gastric vessels
No. 4sa	LN along the short gastric vessels
No. 4sb	LN along the left gastroepiploic vessels
No. 4d	LN along the right gastroepiploic vessels
No. 5	Suprapyloric LN
No. 6	Infrapyloric LN
No. 7	LN along the left gastric artery
No. 8a	LN along the common hepatic artery (anterosuperior group)
No. 8b	LN along the common hepatic artery (posterior group)
No. 9	LN along the celiac artery
No. 10	LN at the splenic hilum
No. 11p	LN along the proximal splenic artery
No. 11d	LN along the distal splenic artery
No. 12a	LN in the hepatoduodenal ligament (along the hepatic artery)
No. 12b	LN in the hepatoduodenal ligament (along the bile duct)
No. 12p	LN in the hepatoduodenal ligament (behind the portal vain)
No. 13	LN on the posterior surface of the pancreatic head
No. 14v	LN along the superior mesenteric vein
No. 14a	LN along the superior mesenteric artery
No. 15	LN along the middle colic vessels
No. 16a1	LN in the aortic hiatus
No. 16a2	LN around the abdominal aorta (from the upper margin of the celiac trunk to the lower margin of the left renal vein)
No. 16b1	LN around the abdominal aorta (from the lower margin of the left renal vein to the upper margin of the inferior mesenteric artery)
No. 16b2	LN around the abdominal aorta (from the upper margin of the inferior mesenteric artery to the aortic bifurcation)
No. 17	LN on the anterior surface of the pancreas head
No. 18	LN along the inferior margin on the pancreas
No. 19	Infradiaphragmatic LN
No. 20	LN in the esophageal hiatus of the diaphragm
No. 110	Paraesophageal LN in the lower thorax
No. 111	Supradiaphragmatic LN
No. 112	Posterior mediastinal LN

Table 2: Regional lymph nodes for Gastric Adenocarcinoma Node Staging

The most commonly used classification supported by the UICC (International Union for Cancer Control) and used in western countries requires a minimum of 15 evaluated nodes for an adequate staging (Edge, 2010, Kim, 2001, Roder 1998). It is based in the TNM staging that is revised periodically according with understanding of the cancer prognosis and the last edition was presented in 2009 and published in 2009 (Sobin et al, 2009, Edge, 2010). It uses a wide datasets from Europe, Asia and United States allowing emerging evidence to support changes in the cancer-staging criteria. Moreover this new edition of the UICC-TNM staging manual considers that tumors arising at the esophagogastric junction (EGJ) or arising in the proximal 5 cm of the stomach (cardia) that extends into the EGJ or esophagus are staged using the TNM system for the adenocarcinoma of the esophagus. Although it is based in an extended datasets of patients that underwent surgical resection of the tumor, the TNM classification may not have a determinant efficacy after neoadjuvant chemotherapy and it is based essentially on the number of affected lymph nodes rather than their location or significance.

MDCT is one of the preferred methods to undergo preoperative TNM staging, evaluation of resectability and control of GA (Shinohara 2005 et al, NCCN Guidelines.2010, Patnana, 2011). It is an accessible and relatively cheap technique with recent developments such as thin collimation images, near-isotropic voxel acquisitions, multiplanar reformations (MPR), and virtual endoscopy. Technical refinement as a variant designed hydro-MDCT with air and water distention of the stomach, may allow virtual gastroscopy images to analyze endoluminal disease and superior differentiation of tumor tissue from the rest of the wall of the organ. MDCT performed with dynamic contrast-enhanced images, represents a robust alternative or complement to EUS in preoperative T and N staging (Habermann , 2004). This investigator compared CT with EUS in the preoperative staging of GA of 51 patients with T2 to T4 disease, obtaining a correct T and N staging of 76% and 70% for CT and 86% and 90% for EUS,; such differences were not statistically significant with a p value of 0.55 for T staging and 0.99 for N staging. Likewise, Hwang et al (2010) in a series of 271 patients obtained an efficacy in T and N staging of 76,6% and 62,8% for CT and 74,7% and 66% for EUS.

Such results have been possible with the implementation of the multidetector technology with multiple acquisitions, near-isotropic imaging and high quality of MPR.

Accordingly, the study protocol must include water distention, as a neutral (iso-density contrast agent) (Horton 2000, 2003) or negative contrast agent in order to avoid the interference of a positive intraluminal contrast agent with the contrast-enhanced effect of the intravenous contrast (Horton 2000, 2003) or a false lesion effect caused by incomplete dissolution of the contrast agent inside the stomach (Winter et al, 1996). Moreover, a negative contrast agent like air using effervescent granules is more effective for gastroscopic evaluation allowing better detectability for T-staging of GC compared to the water distention technique (Park et al, 2010). Using a hypotonic agent might be considered an option considering the short interval of time of images acquisition and the somewhat erroneous interpretation of peristaltic gastric waves in the tumoral area.

There are different positions available depending on the location of the tumor and the used oral contrast and supine positions are the most used ones. With a negative contrast like air, a left posterior oblique position (LPO) provides better visualization of the lower third of the stomach. On the contrary, the right lateral decubitus provides better distention of the upper third and may diminish the obscureness of the lesion by interference from proper lumen-wall interface caused by the use of effervescent granules and residual water (Kim et al, 2005). Water is used as a neutral or negative intraluminal contrast material and should be administered gradually in an amount superior to 750 ml, with half of the dose immediately before the beginning of the examination. Such procedure is important to eliminate small air bubbles beneath the level of water and to assure the gastric distention. The administration of effervescent granule is an optional step that increases the volume of distended stomach and may be used for gastric virtual endoscopy offering further information concerning the mucosal detail that might be important to delineate small lesions (Lee et al, 2012).

The usual imaging pattern of the normal gastric wall in a contrast-enhanced study allows the identification of three distinct layers (Meyers, 2000, Hargunami et al, 2009). These layers are an internal hyperdense contrast-enhancing layer representing the mucosal layer, an intermediate low attenuation stripe, representing the submucosa and an outermost layer demonstrating intermediate enhancement, representing the muscularis propria and the serosa.

Identification of parietal compromise by gastric malignant lesions may allow an evaluation of its mural extent. The early arterial phase and the venous phase of contrast enhancement are considered useful for the delineation of small lesions like precocious tumors already mentioned and called "early cancers" (Mani et al, 2001, Takao et al, 1998), while the interstitial or equilibrium late phase may be more useful in the evaluation of more advanced mural lesions because of tumor-induced fibrosis (Takao et al, 1998). Small lesions may be more difficult to delineate or even non-visualized by MDCT and the majority of such lesions are early cancers without regional lymph node metastasis (Yu et al, 2007).

New multidetector row CT scanners with near-isotropic imaging and MPR give way to several plane reformations, usually coronal, sagittal or perpendicular to the long axis of tumors for better delineation of their relationship to adjacent structures. Some authors registered high efficacy of MDCT staging by the use of tridimensional reformations (Kim et al 2009, Chen et al, 2007). Reformations may be obtained also with other techniques like "volume rendering", depicting an image with endoscopic effect (virtual endoscopy) that is useful to depict gastric rugae or small lesions (Horton, 2003), or through the technique of vessel-probe (Moschetta et al, 2010) with an even higher efficiency in the T staging of the lesions.

Intravenous contrast material should be low-osmolarity and nonionic in order to diminish the possibility of adverse reactions that might preclude or make the examination unreadable. The administrated volume and concentrations ranges between 100 and 150 ml and 30 to 35% of iodine concentration with an automatic injection device at a rate of 2 to 5 ml/s. A 20-40 ml flush of saline serum may be done after the injection of the contrast material to increment its contrast effect.

Most recently published data about GC imaging is based in the staging criteria of the 6th edition of the AJCC. With this classification T1 was diagnosed by abnormal vascularity of the superficial gastric wall, T2 by global compromise of the gastric wall without significant modification of the external contour, T3 by alteration of the external contour with increased densification of adjacent peri-gastric fat and T4 by loss of cleavage plan to adjacent organs (D´Elia et al, 2000, Kumano et al, 2005, Lim et al, 2006). With the new 7th edition of the UICC classification the criteria may be modified to different stages with previous T2 changing to T3, previous T3 changing to T4A and previous T4 changing to T4B. With MDCT the detectability of T1 tumors is low and T1a and T1b may not be possible to differentiate each other with EUS being a better technique to differentiate T1a form T1b tumors (Hwang et al, 2010). Similar results were determined by Lee et al (2010) although emphasizing the potential role of MDCT as a preoperative tool in local staging of EGC and to plan the optimal treatment for patients.

As mentioned before, T1 and T2 of the more recent UICC classification may be considered with a low probability of metastatic lymph node disease when the lesion is not seen with MDCT (Yu et al, 2007). Shimizu et al (6) found also a low percentage of EGC identified by state-of-the art MDCT (14 cases of a series of 41 patients) with a detection rate of 17 and 69% for mucosal and submucosal involvement (Figure 3). Since most cases of EGC may be of non-protruded type (Yu et al, 2007), MDCT with gastric water distention may not be the best method for its diagnosis even with thin slices and MPR. The abnormal contrast-enhancement of mucosal lesions may difficult to distinguish from normal mucosal enhancement and to differentiate between a T1 or T2 lesion may be difficult if the normal three layer pattern is not identified (Takao et al, 1998). Furthermore, it may be a problem to differentiate between the compromise of the serosa, actually staged as T3, and its rupture, currently staged as T4A (Bandhari 2004, Habermann et al,2004).

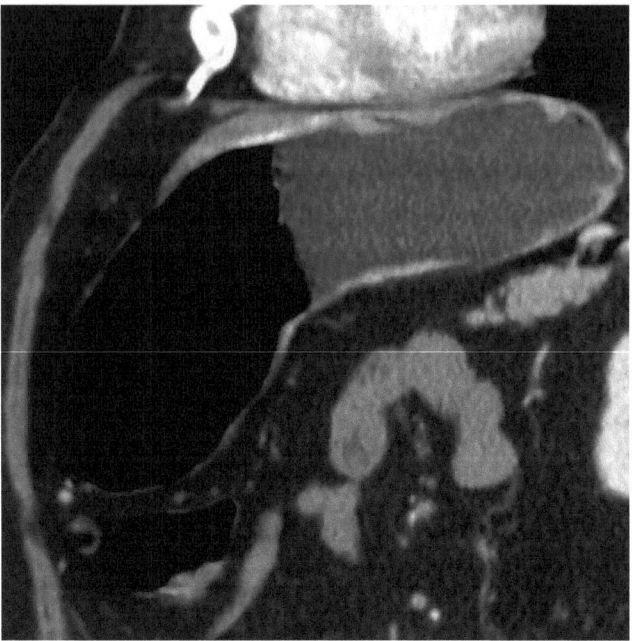

Figure 3

Figure 3: Normal study in a patient with early gastric cancer. Sagittal reconstructions revealing normal appearance of the gastric wall in a patient with diagnosed adenocarcinoma (15 mm tubular adenoma with high-grade dysplasia, located in the posterior wall of the body).

The degree and pattern of contrast enhancement may be influenced by the histological characterization of GA. Undifferentiated (Kumano et al, 2005, Takao et al, 1985), scirrhous and fibrotic tumors may be better seen in delayed interstitial phase or their enhancement may be similar or not differentiated from the entire normal gastric wall during the early or delayed phases (Lee et al, 2000)

Lymph node compromise by malignant tissue is another challenging task of TNM staging by imaging, according with the low accuracy of non aggressive imaging methods in the evaluation of lymphatic micro-metastasis (Patnana, 2010). For instance a prospective study revealed a significant difference between the mean diameter of non involved regional nodes (4,1 mm) versus involved regional lymph nodes (6mm) and 55% of the malignant lymph nodes measured less than 5 mm (Monig et al, 1999). One of the commonest staging criteria is the lymph node size and the used upper limits of the normal size may vary between 6 mm and 8mm in the short-axis diameter (D´Elia et al, 2000, Shinohara et al 2005, Hur et al, 2006, Hwang et al, 2010, Pan et al, 2010). Determining the size of the largest visualized lymph node (both long-axis and short-axis diameter) may give an accuracy for N staging of GC comparable to the traditional method of counting the total of considered positive nodes (Yan et al, 2010) and nodal counts can be used as a surrogate marker for surgical curability of gastric cancer (Kawaguchi, 2012)

Other criteria to be considered are: a) distance from the enlarged node to the tumor (N1 if nearer than 3 cm or N2 if more distant than 3 cm, Pan et al, 2010), b) clustered small lymph nodes or stranding of peri-nodal tissues (Chen 2007), c) contrast enhancement superior to 85 HU (Chen et al, 2010, Fukuya et al, 1995) or 100 HU (Shinohara et al, 2005) and d) lymph node necrosis.

There are few references about the effect on neoadjuvant chemotherapy on MDCT GA imaging and its concomitant effect in the restaging of the tumor gastric cancer research (Park et al, 2008, Lee et al, 2009) or comparing the 6th edition versus the 7th edition of the UICC TNM classification (Kawagushi et al, 2011). Different results may be seen with MDCT staging after neoadjuvant chemotherapy (Figure 3) with a trend to overstaging compared to preoperative staging without chemotherapy (Lee et al, 2009) or to understaging compared to surgical pathological analysis (Park et al, 2008). Histological tumor regression grade is an objective measure of the effects of neoadjuvant chemotherapy in GA. Other features that might be evaluated by MDCT are vascular changes including organizing thrombi in the perigastric adipose tissue or marked transmural fibrosis in the area of the tumor bed (Becker et al, 2003). These features may affect staging under the neoadjuvant chemotherapy effect and should not be confused with progression of the disease or deficient response to chemotherapy.

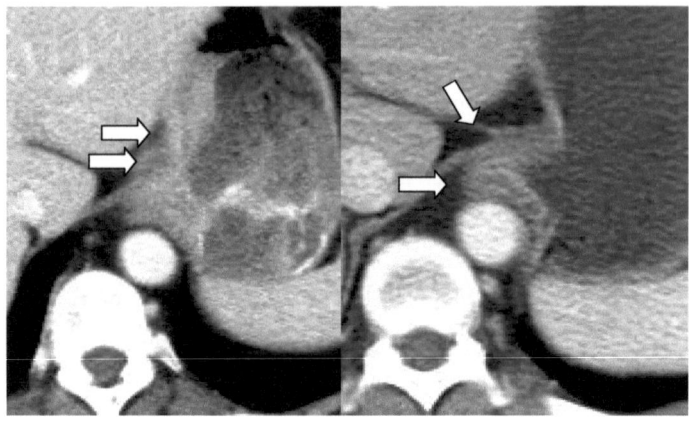

Figure 4

Figure 4 A (left) and B (right): Example of GA after neoadjuvant chemotherapy. Extensive lesion staged as T4A (image left, white arrows) that underwent neoadjuvant chemotheraphy with a post-operative stage of T1b N0 (image right, white arrows)

Considering the mentioned limitations regarding the evaluation of metastatic lymph node disease and tumoral evaluation after neoadjuvant chemotherapy and the advances obtained with state of the art MDCT the purposes of our work are:

a) to compare the efficacy of Computed Tomography technology by MDCT through an accessible protocol for T and N staging of GA in patients that underwent surgical resection with curative intention.

b) to analyze the impact of some important pathologic characteristics in cases of significant discrepancy between pathologic and imaging results, in order to introduce a compensation or surrogate factor or marker to a better staging of nodal compromise.

Material and Methods

A retrospective study with the accordance of the multidisciplinary cancer group of our institution but without the submission of approval by the institutional review board was performed. Between January 2010 and July 2012, available patient files retrieved from the Radiology, Surgery and Pathology Departments Archiving Systems to compare the results of surgical pathology with previous CT scans (performed less than sixty days before surgery). One hundred sixty nine patients underwent partial or total gastrectomy and lymphadenectomy D2/D3 for gastric neoplasms and sixty-nine of those were included in our study according the following criteria: a) MDCT performed at our institution, including gastric water distention and at least one of the three usual post-contrast phases (arterial, venous or interstitial), sixty four patients, b) non contrast enhanced CT associated with MRI performed in the same day (3 patients), c) Computed Tomography performed with helical technology (2 patients), d) all studies were performed less than sixty days before surgical intervention and had a positive endoscopic diagnosis of gastric adenocarcinoma.

Standard multi-detector CT was performed with a 16 Channel or a 64 Channel Scanner. Patients were informed of the indications and drawbacks of CT iodinated intravenous study but an informed consent was waived. Oral preparation included fasting for 4 to 6 h and the ingestion of tap water, between 750 and 1000 ml (hydro-CT technique) with 5 g of effervescent granules to increase the gastric distention in the case of hydro-CT, or contrast-positive oral agent in the previous 20 to 40 minutes (two patients). Images were performed in the arterial and portal phase after injection of 80 to 120 ml of iodine in the concentration of 300 to 320 mg/ml, with an average speed of 2cc/second and followed by a posterior 40 cc saline bolus with the same flow rate.

Used CT scanners were a 16-detector row (Brightspeed S; GE; Healthcare, Milwaukee, WI, USA) or a 64-detector row CT scanner (LightSpeed VCT; GE Healthcare, Milwaukee, WI, USA). Two sets of CT scans were obtained. Unenhanced CT was generally not performed. For contrast-enhanced CT, a dose of 2 ml/kg of a non-ionic contrast agent (Iopromide, Ultravist; Schering, Berlin, Germany) was

23

administrated intravenously through an 18-gauge angiographic catheter at a rate of 2ml/s using a power injector (OptiVantage, Liebel-Flarsheim; Mallinckrodt, Neustadt, Germany). First CT scanning was started 40 s after contrast material injection (in the arterial phase). The scanning range was from the xyphoid process to the lower end of the stomach. Then a second set of CT scanning was started 70 s after contrast material injection (in the portal venous phase) from the diaphragm to the pubis.

Usual CT scanning parameters were as follows for 64 detector rows: beam collimation, 0.625/1.25mm/20–40 mm (or 10-20 mm with 16 rows); pitch, 0.984; kVp/effective mA, 120/until 300; gantry rotation time, 0.8 s. Isotropic raw data were acquired with a slice thickness of 1.25 mm and an interval of 1.25 mm at MDCT. Using this raw data, a transverse image was obtained with a slice thickness of 3.75 mm and an interval of 3.75 mm, then coronal and occasionally sagittal or oblique MPR images were reconstructed on a workstation. Each MPR image was obtained at 3/4-mm intervals with a slice thickness of 3/4 mm.

Analysis of images: studies were evaluated and classified in consensus by three radiologists with different experience in abdominal imaging (respectively one consultant with twenty years of experience in abdominal imaging and more than two hundred cases of gastric cancer evaluation by CT or MRI, one assistant with fifteen years of experience in abdominal imaging and a third assistant with ten years of experience in abdominal imaging).

Individual staging of each case was obtained by consensus between two of the three considered readers. Because the aim was to ascertain CT efficacy in tumor and nodal staging and to develop a robust staging system by imaging the involved radiologists were not blind to the surgical staging of each individual case, previous information of the endoscopic evaluation and consequent localization of the lesion was available in every cases.

CT T and N staging was done through source axial images or axial, coronal, sagittal or oblique reconstructions, using the following criteria;

T staging:

-T1: unseen lesion or lesion with superficial irregularity or contrast enhancement or thickening, sparing the intermediate hypodense submucosal area.

-T2: identifiable lesion with partial or almost total obliteration of the intermediate post-contrast hypodense wall and a regular contour of the external gastric layer.

-T3: total compromise of the gastric wall with a regular or minimally irregular external contour (not exceeding 5 mm).

-T4A: transmural lesions with irregular external contour superior to 5 mm in length or with a fat soft tissue stranding.

-T4B: transmural lesion with loss of cleavage plan to an adjacent organ namely the diaphragmatic crux, left lobe of the liver or pancreas.

N Staging: each of the following criteria were considered synonymous with an involved lymph node:

-lymph node with a biggest short-axis superior to 7 mm. Such short axis was measured with a cursor in the transverse plan or coronal/sagittal plane when a larger short axis diameter was evaluated by such reformations.

-lymph node with a short axis equal or smaller than 7 mm but revealing a measurement of region of interest superior to 80 Hounsfield Units (HU) in one area superior to 0,10 cm2 or a lymph node revealing central necrosis.

-area of nodular or stranded densities less than 5 cm away from the main lesion or a conglomerate of three or more nodes equal or smaller than 7 mm of short axis was considered an additional criteria for lymph node involvement.

-overall diminished fat cleavage plans between the stomach, pancreas and less omentun was considered a pattern of N3B involvement (besides T4B staging).

The considered criteria were added and the final number was considered the number of involved lymph nodes with subsequent nodal staging according with the recently revised UICC criteria of the 7th edition (N0: no nodes involved, N1: one or two nodes involved, N2: three to six nodes involved, N3A: seven to fifteen nodes involved and N3B: more than fifteen nodes involved).

Data were compared with surgical staging obtained by total or partial gastrectomy with curative intention in order to evaluate efficacy in T and N staging.

Evaluation of MDCT efficacy in regional or distant metastatic disease was outside the scope of this study.

Since all patients had a positive previous diagnosis of GA by UGE (upper gastrointestinal endoscopy) confirmed by surgery, and tumors not seen by CT were staged by imaging as T1 tumors, there were no true negatives for global T staging in this series. For a global evaluation of T staging, sensitivity was measured considering overstaged patients as false-positives and understaged patients as false-negatives. Additionally a separate evaluation of true positive, true negative, false positive or false negative for each stage was performed for N and T staging. In this case correct staging was considered a true positive, overstaging by imaging was considered false-positive and understaging false negative; all other cases of the table were considered true negatives for the analyzed T or N stage. Values were obtained for each stage dividing parameters obtained by the number of cases and a final score was determined by the average of summation of each stage.

The personal experience and the literature data (Hur et al, 2006, Park et al, 2008, Yan et al, 2010) point out the inaccuracy of MDCT for nodal staging with a trend to understaging in the pre-operative evaluation due to inability to diagnose micro-metastasis and to differentiate between a metastatic or reactive node. To compensate these limitations some prognostic items were subsequently analyzed in the diagnostic imaging in the case of major discrepancy of results for T and N staging (inaccurate diagnostic staging superior to correct diagnostic staging) and if the number of patients in question was superior to 20 % of patients evaluated (at least fourteen patients of a total of sixty nine). The prognostic factors evaluated was respectively the number of nodes considered involved, the deepness of the tumor extension, and the type of tumor histology according the Lauren Classification, three considered factors of prognostic significance in the natural history of GA. The deepness of tumor extension is the basis of T staging and the number of involved nodes the basis of N staging. The Lauren classification has been demonstrated to be an independent prognostic factor (Polkowski et al, 1999) and influencing the patient survival (Marreli et al, 2002).

The rationale of this procedure is to find out a presumption or surrogate factor that may improve and help the accuracy of MDCT staging of the disease. The incidence of the prognostic factors in data corresponding to true positives of the considered stage was compared with incidence of prognostic factors in discrepant data (inaccurate diagnostic staging corresponding to a higher or lower pathologic staging) to confirm or exclude such prognostic factors as potential presumptive or surrogate factors for a more accurate T or N staging of the disease.

Results

The correlation between the diagnostic studies and the surgical specimens for depth of wall invasion (T) and nodal (N) staging are shown in Table 3 and Table 4:

Table 3: T staging correlation between MDCT/CT and Surgery for Gastric Adenocarcinoma in sixty nine patients (*)

T Staging Pathology	T1 (11)	T2 (13)	T3 (23)	T4A (18)	T4B (4)
Radiology					
T1 (7)	7	0	0	0	0
T2 (8)	3	4	0	1	0
T3 (31)	1	8	20	2	
T4A (17)	0	1	3	12	1
T4B (6)	0	0	0	3	3

(*) Data are number of patients

27

Table 4: N staging correlation between MDCT/CT and Surgery for Gastric
Adenocarcinoma in sixty nine patients (*)

N Staging Pathology	N0 (23)	N1 (10)	N2 (12)	N3A (18)	N3B (6)
Radiology					
N0 (21)	16	3	2	0	0
N1 (17)	7	5	3	0	2
N2 (25)	0	2	7	14	2
N3A (4)	0	0	0	4	0
N3B (2)	0	0	0	0	2

(*) Data are numbers of patients

Overall sensitivity obtained for T was 92 % and overall sensitivity and specificity obtained for N staging was 40,9 % and 64 %. There was an agreement for T staging in 46 patients (66,7 %) and for N staging in 34 patients (49,3 %). As every patients have a confirmed diagnosis of GA and lesions not seen on MDCT were considered stage T1, there were no true negative cases and overall specificity for T staging was not evaluated.

Separate evaluation of sensitivity and specificity for each T stage and overall addition of results divided by the number of patients were: 93,3 % sensitivity and 92,9 % specificity for T staging and 61,2 % sensitivity and 95,1 % specificity for N staging (Tables 5 and 6).

Table 5: Separate evaluation of T Staging Sensitivity and Specificity

T Staging	Number of patients	Stage Sensitivity(%)	Stage Specificity(%)
T1	11	100	93,5
T2	13	100	86,2
T3	23	100	93,9
T4A	18	80	94,4
T4B	4	75	100
Total averaged	69	93,3	92,9

Table 6: Separate evaluation of N Staging Sensitivity and Specificity

N Staging	Number of patients	Stage Sensitivity(%)	Stage Specificity(%)
N0	23	100	86,8
N1	10	62,5	96,7
N2	12	58,3	100
N3A	18	22,2	100
N3B	6	33,3%	100
Total averaged	69	61,2	95,1

Considering the results obtained for N staging there was a low sensibility for N3A due to 14 false negatives (fourteen patients staged as N2 instead of N3A). The analysis of the prognostic factors mentioned in the section of Material and Methods is presented in Table 7, including patients with diagnostic N2 disease, where patients 1 to 14 correspond to false negative diagnostic N2 Staging of pathologic correct staging N3A and patients 15 to 21 correspond to true positive diagnostic N2 Staging.

Table 7: List of patients with diagnostic N2 Staging and N3A/N2 pathologic staging (N3A patients 1 to 14 and N2 patients 15 to 21)

Patients Series	Number of metastatic lymph nodes	T Staging	Lauren´s Classification
1	4	4 B	Difuse
2	3	4 A	Intestinal
3	3	4 A	Difuse
4	3	3	Difuse
5	3	4 A	Intestinal
6	3	3	Difuse
7	3	4 B	Intestinal
8	3	3	Difuse
9	4	4 A	Intestinal
10	3	3	Intestinal
11	3	4 B	Intestinal
12	4	3	Intestinal
13	4	4 A	Mixed
14	3	3	Diffuse

15	5	4 A	Mixed
16	3	3	Mixed
17	3	3	Intestinal
18	4	3	Intestinal
19	3	3	Mixed
20	3	3	Intestinal
21	3	3	Diffuse

Comparing data between patients 1 to 14 and 15 to 21 it stands out that eight of nine patients with a T Staging level 4 had a N stage level 3 A with a T 4 staging difference between both groups. The difference of T4 incidence in these two groups was statistically different (p: 0.039%) according to McNemar´s Test, an adequate test to evaluate the differences of two dichotomous variables in a two for two cross-tabulation when series are subjected to different situations (Bland, 2009). The differences of incidence of Diffuse type of Lauren´s classification between both groups did not change sensibility and specificity in the same magnitude.

Considering patients with MDCT staging T4 N 2 as changing N staging to level N3A, the overall sensibility and specificity of N staging changes to 58,1 and 61,5 % and the accuracy (agreement) to 59,4% respectively (Table 8, 9 and 10).

Table 9 shows values of N Staging accuracy sensitivity and specificity for the overall author´s series (AS) and after surrogate factor of T4 disease (AS/T4) for major differences of staging in the case of diagnostic N2 disease, and surrogate factor of Diffuse type of Lauren´s Classification in the same patients.

Diagnosis of N3B disease is also a challenge with a sensitivity of 33,3% (two of six patients correctly staged). Of these patients four belonged to the mixed type and two to the diffuse type of Lauren Classification. In two cases MPR reconstructions were not accessible and five patients had lesions larger than 8 cm.

Results obtained in accuracy of MDCT/CT in T staging has been compared with other series (Chen,2007, D´Elia 2007, Park 2010) and revealed only statistically relevant difference for Chen´s Series evaluated by MPR (Fisher´s exact test p-value of 0.004). For N Staging (Table 10), most differences were statistically significant without the use of T4 Staging as a Surrogate factor for diagnostic N2 Staging (Chen 2007, D´Elia 2007, Habermann 2007, Pan 2010). With such surrogate only Chen´s series with MPR revealed a significant difference (Fisher´s exact test p-value of 0.034).

Table 8: N Staging with surrogate factor T4 changing T4/N2 diagnosis to T4/N3A diagnosis (*)

N Staging	Pathology	N0(23)	N1 (10)	N2 (12)	N3A (18)	N3B (6)
Radiology						
N0 (21)		16	3	2	0	0
N1 (17)		7	5	3	0	2
N2 (16)		0	2	6	6	2
N3A (13)		0	0	1	12	0
N3B (2)		0	0	0	0	2

(*) Data are number of patients

Table 9: Accuracy, Sensitivity and Specificity of N Staging without and with Surrogate Factors

T4 and Diffuse type of Lauren´s Classification (*)

N Staging	Accuracy	Sensitivity	Specificity
Author's series (AS)	49,3	40,9	65,4
AS with T4 Surrogate to change N2 to N3A	59,4	58,1	61,5
AS with Diffuse type Surrogate to change N2 to N3A	56,5	53,4	61,5

(*) Data are in percentages

Table 10: Comparison of accuracy, sensitivity and specificity between our series with Surrogate

T4 factor (AS/T4) and data from the literature (*)

N Staging	Accuracy	Sensitivity	Specificity
Chen (Transv.), 2006	71	71,4	70
Chen (MPR), 2006	78	86	65
Habermann, 2004	70	73	66,7
D´Elia,2000	71	74,6	63,8
AS/T4	59,4	58,1	61,5

(*) Data are in percentages

Discussion

One of the main indications of CT in the evaluation of GA is to determine surgical resectability by excluding metastatic disease and recent developments as using oral negative contrast agent, gastric distention, dynamic contrast-enhancement and MPR have improved the potential of this technique (Hargunami et al, 2009, Park et al, 2010).

In our study, results obtained with MDCT/CT in T staging revealed only statistically relevant difference for Chen´s Series evaluated by MPR (Fisher´s exact test two-sided p-value of 0.004) (Chen et al, 2006, D´Elia et al, 2000, Pan et al, 2010, Park et al, 2010). For N Staging, most differences were statistically significant without the use of T4 Staging as a Surrogate factor for diagnostic N2 Staging (Chen et al, 2006, D´Elia et al, 2000, Habermann et al, 2004, Pan et al, 2010). With such surrogate only Chen´s series with MPR revealed a significant difference with Fisher´s exact test (two-size p-value: 0.034). Such results must take into consideration the accessibility of the protocol that influences the robustness of the examination. Indeed, using of a lower dose of intravenous contrast, lower speed of intravenous injection or the exclusion of the administration of intravenous hypotonic agent may justify an overall lower sensitivity for N staging (40,9 %) and a less high accuracy for T staging (66,7 %); furthermore our methodology considered five grades of involvement for T staging and four levels of involvement for N staging that added further exigency to the imaging efficacy (Park et al, 2010, Lee et al, 2012).

The known limitations of MDCT in T and N staging justified to adopt a compensation or surrogate factor for N staging, with a positive influence in the accuracy of the method. That was recently demonstrated by Kawaguchi (2012) in a series of 92 patients were a nodal count of four or more metastatic lymph nodes was demonstrated to have a sensitivity of 94,4% and a specificity of 71,6% to distinguish curative from non curative patients.

Unseen lesions are considered to have a low probability of metastatic disease and are predominantly lesions involving the mucosa (Yu et al, 2007). Result in our series was consistent with these concepts, since there were only three unseen lesions (Figure 3), all of them classified as T1 lesions confined to the mucosa. Only one of those six patients classified with T1 disease had metastatic N1 disease (a lesion that was detected by MDCT and belonged to the diffuse type of Lauren´s classification). Additionally one of such unseen tumors was even not macroscopically visible.

There were four false positives for diagnosing T1 disease and two corresponded to studies without intravenous contrast and complemented by MRI, where the mural enhancement was not evaluated; a third cased corresponded to one contrast enhanced study without significant gastric distention that diminished the conspicuity of the lesion. If such cases were excluded from the series the efficacy for T1 staging would be increased. These data suggest a high accuracy for T1 evaluation with MDCT even without significant iodine dose or speed of contrast injection, although there was not the pretension to differentiate T1A form T1B lesions and considering that high contrast enhancement of superficial gastric lesions may be a requisite for their detection. Otherwise the over- or under-staging of T1 and T2 lesions may have a limited effect in the decision for a curative resection.

Differentiation between T2 and T3 disease is more difficult by MDCT and our series showed 9 false positive cases (overstaging) for T2 evaluation (Figure 5); in two cases patients underwent neoadjuvant chemotherapy that may increase the fibrotic component of the wall and hence misleading mural evaluation (Lee et al, 2009, Ng et al, 1998). The relative limitation of our protocol concerning the iodine concentration, volume or speed of injection may justify the difficult differentiation between the lower density intermediate zone representing the submucosa and the intermediate density outer layer representing the muscularis propria and the serosa. That was not such a problem in the previous staging of the 6th edition of UICC and may deserve further investigation according with the implementation of the current classification.

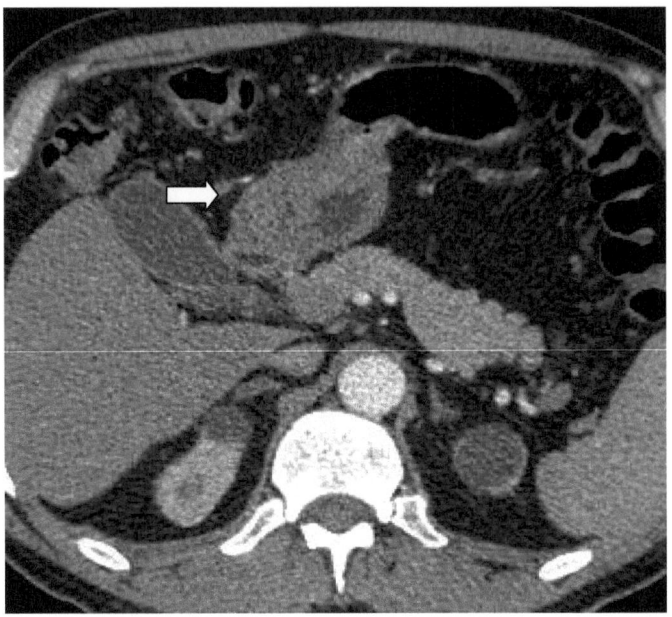

Figure 5

Figure 5: Example of GC Pathologic T Stage T2 and diagnostic T stage T3. Anterior neoplasm of antrum (white arrow) revealing an heterogeneous thickened wall with regular external contour. Diagnostic T staging was T3, mainly because of the tumour size, while Pathology revealed T2 cancer.

The evaluation of advanced stages of mural disease was adequate for T3, T4A and T4B lesions (Figure 6). T3 lesions may reveal some irregularity of the external contour that may be caused by inflammatory reaction or tumor extension difficult to differentiate each other, particularly in wasted patients with a reduced perigastric fat deposition. The difference of enhancement between the arterial, portal or interstitial phase was not considered a criterion for such differentiation (Pan et al, 2003). MDCT allows excellent MPR that can be useful for a superior delineation of the external contour and the relationship of the organ with adjacent structures and the interspersed fat plans (Chen et al, 2007).

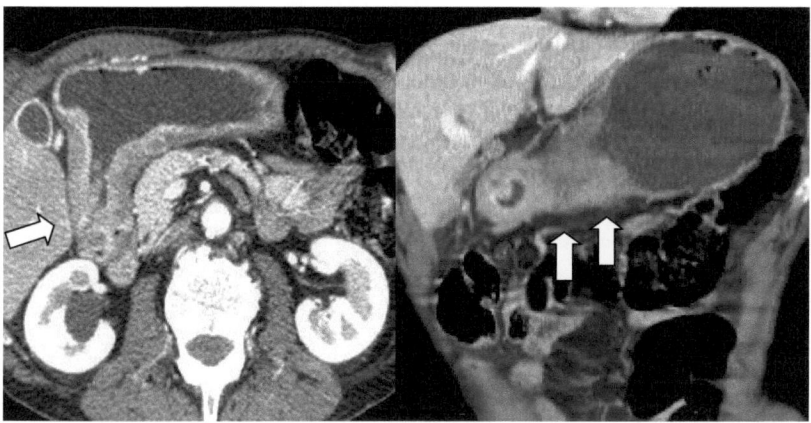

Figure 6

Figure 6 A (left) and B (right): Example of T4A GC. Mixed poor differentiated gastric adenocarcinoma with T4A imaging staging (slight irregular external contour in the lower border of the antrum, white arrows in the right; tumour also shown in the left, white arrow).

To use the disappearance of the fat cleavage plan between the gastric lesion and the adjacent organs may be misleading (Fukuya et al, 1997) and it is clinically useful to consider more than one grade of infiltration surrounding the stomach and loss of fat plan interface (Pan et al, 2003). Limitations related with spatial and contrast resolution or partial-volume effects still limit the assessment of microscopic invasion of the pancreatic capsule or the left liver lobe (D´Elia et al, 2000).

It is well known the inability of CT to detect micrometastases and metastatic involvement of small nodes because of the considered limitations with partial volume artifacts, noise and resolution; moreover larger nodes with contrast-enhancement may be caused by metastatic involvement or reactive hyperplasia (Figure 7) and contrast enhancement is difficult to evaluate in small nodes. Using the seventh edition of the UICC classification is an additional challenge namely for staging advanced nodal disease. Likewise Kawagushi et al, (2011) demonstrated better correlation of lymph nodes metastasis with the 13th JCGC staging system than with the seventh edition of the UICC TNM classification (Sobin et al, 2010) and a significant difference between the number of metastatic nodes diagnosed by MDCT and pathology.

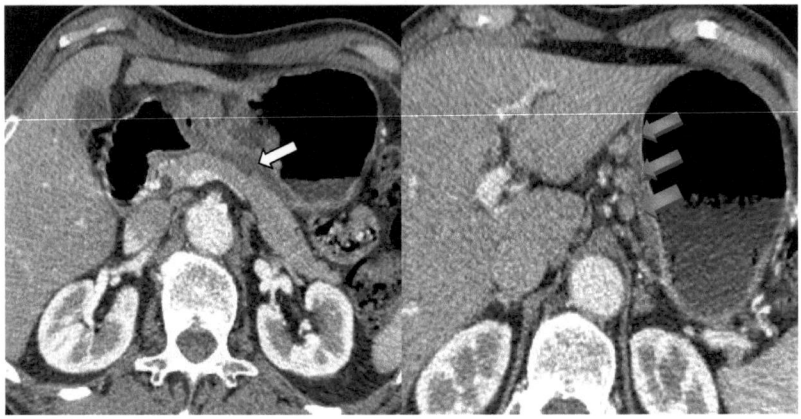

Figure 7

Figure 7 A (left) and B (right): Example of enlarged nodes simulating malignancy. Extensive lesion in the body and antrum with hypodense external contour (white arrow). Imaging and pathological T staging were both T2 while imaging N staging was N2 due to four enlarged nodes in the lesser curvature (green arrows). However pathologic staging after surgery did not reveal malignant nodes (Pathologic staging N0).

The overall accuracy for correct nodal staging reflects the difficulty to measure or evaluate more than six metastatic lymph nodes with the presented criteria. There was a significant difference in accuracy for staging advanced and non-advanced nodal compromise (N3 disease versus N0 to N2 disease. The overall resulting accuracy, sensibility and specificity of 49,3 %, 40,9 % and 64%, improved to values as 59,4%, 58,1% and 61,5% if an additional staging criterion was used (T4 Staging accompanying diagnosed N2 disease as a criterion to increase diagnostic N staging to N3A) (Figure 8).

Our results are included in the lower range of literature results considering that most of the published literature dedicated to T and N staging of GA still use the sixth edition of the AJCC or UICC (Sobin, 2002). Accordingly the sensitivity and specificity obtained for N3A was 22 and 100%, different from the values obtained by Chen et al (2007) of 43 and 92 % with transverse images and 72 and 94% with MPRs and 74,3 % and 91,7 % obtained by Pan et al (2010) where the same number of involved nodes (7 to 15) were staged according with the 6h Edition of TNM staging of the UICC as N2. However, with the correction or compensation factor of classifying as N3A cases, initially diagnosed N2 patients that presented T staging of level T4, values of sensibility and specificity in N3A staging changed to 66,6% and 100% respectively and were not different from the ones presented by the mentioned investigators.

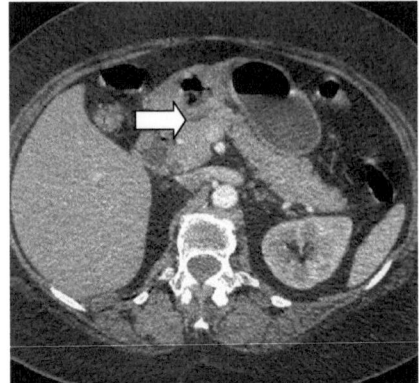

Fig. 8 A

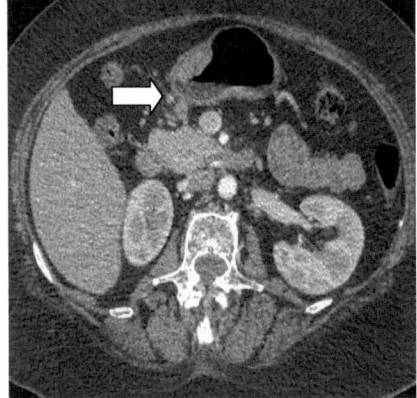

Fig. 8 B

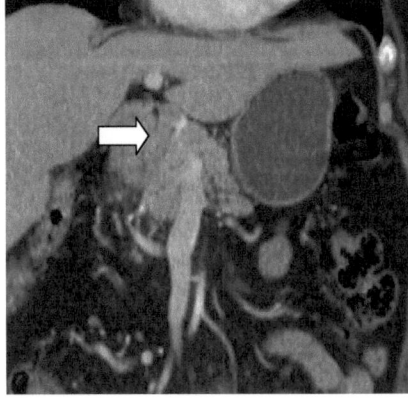

Fig. 8 C

Figure 8 A (top), B (intermediate) and C (bottom): GC with T4 N3A pathologic staging and N2 diagnostic staging. Antral GA causing compression of pancreatic head consistent with T4B staging (Figure 8A, white arrow). Nodal disease (Figure 8B, white arrow) was considered by imaging N2 disease with an enlarged node located inferiorly to the antrum. Pathologic N staging was N3A and the advanced T staging might be a surrogate of more advanced nodal disease. Figure 8C revealing mass effect over the pancreatic head by the antral GA (white arrow).

We also found difficult measuring more than six nodes with a short axis larger than 7 mm, at least in early stages and in the transverse plane (Kawagushi, 2012). The classification of lymph node involvement based in contrast enhancement may be also difficult to obtain mainly in the case of small nodes concerning the effect of volume averaging caused by a larger region of interest and the effect of noise when a very small region of interest was applied. A better quality of measurement of the larger short-axis of every node may be considered although it may be time consuming; a larger volume or concentration of contrast or a faster speed of injection of the contrast media may also influence a possible rise of accuracy with MDCT in this pathology.

The values of sensitivity and specificity for separate N0 staging disease were similar to other series (sensitivity for N0 disease versus N1 and N2 disease with the criteria of the 6th edition of the UICC, in the series of D´Elia, 2000) and sensitivity and specificity for N0 disease in the series of Pan (2010).

For N1 and N2 staging, the results of obtained sensitivity (62,5%:N1 and 58,3%:N2) was slightly lower than values obtained by Pan et al (2010) and Fukuya et al (1995). Kawaguchi (2012) also demonstrated a significant difference of nodal metastatic counts between MDCT and pathology and established an equation to obtain very high sensitivity and specificity in the differentiation between curative and non curative resection.

There was a tendency for MDCT to understage nodal disease (Park et al, 2008, Patnana, 2010, Yan et al, 2010). We believe the main reason should be the inability of CT to diagnose metastatic disease in small lymph nodes and that may be one of the main limitations of our study: there were no measurement of the lymph nodes size by pathology namely the dimensions of the metastatic lymph nodes, wondering if the majority of false-negatives obtained by MDCT were caused by microscopic or metastatic disease in small lymph nodes. This was also true for N3 staging and in our series no patients had more than eight nodes considered positive, even considering the indirect criteria of heterogeneous densification of fat adjacent to the tumor or lack of cleavage plan between superior intra-abdominal organs or in the higher retroperitoneum. Kawagushi et al (2011) also found a significant difference between the number of metastatic nodes diagnosed by imaging and pathology and considered a better correlation of the 13th JCGC staging system with the histological analysis.

There are several limitations in our study. It was a retrospective study with all lesions confirmed by biopsy and known by the panelists and the evaluation was dominated by the opinion of the most experimented radiologist in the area. Furthermore the speed and dose of contrast injection was inferior to the start-of-the-art studies and five patients were not evaluated by MDCT. All this facts isolated or in group could lead to bias. Experience in the MDCT evaluation or staging of patients with GA is a requisite to reduce the inter-observer variability and the final results of the study. The correct evaluation of T and N staging for gastric cancer is time-consuming and requires detail and experience; moreover the correlation with other pathologic data is important as our study suggests. Other limitation concerns about the obtained data which cannot be extrapolated to the general population for a screening purpose were CT performance could be overestimated. The size and location of surgical extracted nodes was not correlated with the interpretation of the imaging data so a node to node correlation was not performed. Nevertheless the routine surgical technique includes a D2 resection (NCCN, 2010) and the majority of unseen nodes were from the perigastric stations with a lesser influence in prognostic and therapeutic perspective.

In conclusion, MDCT T and N staging of GA with a simple, reproducible and accessible protocol allows fairly good levels of accuracy, sensitivity and specificity and such values may be increased in the case of N staging by using a surrogate factor (N3A diagnostic staging in cases of diagnostic N2 disease associated with T4 staging). We also believe that a stricter adherence to the state-of-the-art protocol and a larger clinical experience with GA evaluation may improve the efficiency of GA T and N staging. by MDCT.

Bibliography:

Abdalla E, Pisters P. Staging and preoperative evaluation of upper gastrointestinal malignancies. Semin Oncol. 2004; 31: 513-529.

Bandhari S, Shim CS, Kim JH, et al. Usefulness of three-dimensional, multidetector row CT (virtual gastroscopy and multiplanar reconstruction) in the evaluation of gastric cancer: a comparison with conventional endoscopy, EUS and histopathology. Gastrointestinal Endoscopy. 2004; 59: 619-626.

Ba-Ssalamah A, Prokop M, Uffmann M, et al. (2003) Dedicated multidetector CT of the stomach: spectrum of diseases. Radiographics 23:625–644.

Bastos J, Lunet N, Peleteiro B, et al. Dietary patterns and gastric cancer in a portuguese urban population. Int J Cancer. 2009; 127.433-441.

Becker K, Mueller J, Schulmacher C, Ott K, et al. Histomorphology and Grading of Regression in Gastric Carcinoma Treated with Neoadjuvant Chemotherapy. Cancer 2003; 98: 1521-1530.

Bland M (2009). The analysis of cross-tabulations. In: M. Bland ed. An Introduction to Medical Statistics. 3rd ed. New York, Oxford University Press, 2009. p. 230-255.

Chen CY, Hsu IS, Wu DC, et al. Gastric cancer: Preoperative Local Staging with 3D Multi-detector Row CT-Correlation with Surgical and Histopathologic Results. Radiology. 2007; 242: 472-482.

de Vries AC, Meijer GA, Looman CW, et al. Epidemiological trends of pre-malignant gastric lesions: a long-term nationwide study in the Netherlands. Gut. 2007; 56: 1665-1670.

Dong CX, Deng DJ, Pan KF et al. Promoter methylation of p16 associated with Helicobacter Pylori infection in precancerous gastric lesions: a population-based study. In J Cancer. 2009; 124: 434-439.

D´Elia F, Zingarelli A, Palli D, Grani M. Hydro-dynamic CT preoperative staging of gastric cancer: correlation with pathological findings. A prospective study of 107 cases. Eur Radiol. 2007; 10: 1877-1885.

Edge SB. AJCC cancer staging manual. New York, NY. 7th edition. Springer-Verlag; 2010.

Fenoglio-Preiser CM, Noffsinger AE, Stemmermann GN, et al., eds. The neoplastic stomach in Gastrointestinal pathology: an atlas and text. Philadelphia. Lippincott Williams & Wilkins. 2008.

Fitgerald RC, Caldas C. Clinical implications of E-cadherin associated hereditary diffuse gastric cancer. Gut. 2004; 53: 775-778.

Fukuya T, Honda H, Hayashi T, et al. Lymph node metastases: efficacy for detection with helical CT in patients with gastric cancer. Radiology. 1995; 197: 705–711.

Globocan. Estimated cancer Incidence, Mortality, Prevalence and Disability-adjusted life years (DALYs) Worlwide in 2008. http://globocan.iarc.fr.

Gore RM. Gastric cancer. Clinical and pathologic features. Radiol Clin North Am. 1997; 35: 295–310

Habermann CR, Weiss F, Riecken R, et al. Preoperative staging of gastric adenocarcinoma: comparison of helical CT and endoscopic US. Radiology. 2004; 230(2): 465-471.

Hargunani R, Maclachlan J, Kamiyur S, et al. Cross-sectional imaging of gastric neoplasia. Clin Radiol. 2009; 64: 420-429.

Horton KM, Fishman EK. Current role of CT in imaging of the stomach. RadioGraphics. 2003; 23: 75-87.

Horton KM, Fishman EK. Normal enhancement of the small bowel: evaluation with spiral CT. J Comput Assist Tomogr. 2000; 24: 67-71.

Hur J, Park MS, Lee JH, et al. Diagnostic accuracy of multidetector row computed tomography in T and N staging of gastric cancer with histopathologic correlation. J Comput Assist Tomogr. 2006; 30: 372–377.

Hwang WS, Lee DH, Lee SH, Park YS, Hwang JH, Kim JW, et al. Preoperative staging of gastric cancer by endoscopic ultrasonography and multidetector-row computed tomography. Journal of Gastroenterology and Hepatology. 2010, 25: 512–518.

IARC, 2008. Cited February 3 2011, International Agency of Research on Cancer. Available from
http://globocan.iarc.fr/factsheets/population/factsheet.asp?uno=994

Japanese Gastric Cancer Association, *Japanese Classification of Gastric Cancer.* Tokyo, Japan, Kanehara & Co, 14th edition. 2010.

Japanese Research Society for Gastric Cancer (Japan). The General Rules for the Gastric Cancer Study in Surgery and Pathology (ed. 12). Tokyo. Kanahara Shuppan, 1993.

Kamangar F, Dores GM, Anderson WF. Patterns of cancer incidence, mortality, and prevalence across five continents: defining priorities to reduce cancer disparities in different geographic regions of the world. J Clin Oncol. 2006; 24: 2137–2150.

Katai H, Sano T. Early gastric cancer: concepts, diagnosis, and management. Int J Clin Oncol. 2005; 10: 375–383.

Kawagushi T, Ichikawa D., Komatsu S., Okamoto K. et al. Clinical evaluation of JCGC and TNM Staging on Multidetector-row Computed Tomography in Preoperative Nodal Staging of Gastric Cancer. Hepato-Gastrolenterology. 2011. 58:107-108, Ahead of Print.

Kawagushi T, Komatsu S. Nodal Counts on MDCT as a Surrogate Marker for Surgical Curability in Gastric Cancer. Annals of Surgical Oncology. 2012; 19: 2465-70.

Kim H, Karpeh M, Brennan M. Standardization of the extent of lymphadenectomy for gastric cancer: impact on survival. Advances in Surgery. 2001; 35: 203-223.

Kim HJ, Kim AY, Oh ST, et al. Gastric cancer staging at multi-detector row CT gastrography: comparison of transverse and volumetric CT scanning. Radiology. 2005; 236: 879–885

Kim SH, Lee JM, Han JK, et al. Effect of adjusted positioning on gastric distention and fluid distribution during CT gastrography. Am J Roentgenol. 2005; 185:1180–1184.

Kim JP. Surgical results in gastric cancer. Semin Surg Oncol. 1999; 17: 132–138

Kim YH, Lee KH, Park SH, et al. Staging of T3 and T4 gastric carcinoma with multidetector CT: added value of multiplanar reformations for prediction of adjacent organ invasion. Radiology. 2009; 250: 767-775.

Kumano S., Murakami T., Kim T., Hori M. et al. T Staging of Gastric Cancer: Role of Multi-Detector-Row CT. Radiology. 2005; 237: 961-966.

Kunisaki S, Shimada H, Akiyama H et al. Clinical impact of metastatic lymph node ratio in advanced gastric cancer. Anticancer Res. 2005; 25: 1369-75.

Kwee R, Kwee T. Imaging in local staging of gastric cancer: a systematic review. J Clin Oncol. 2007; 25: 2107-2116.

Ladeiras-Lopes R, Pereira A, Nogueira A et al. Smoking and gastric cancer: systematic review and meta-analysis of cohort studies. Cancer Causes Control. 2008; 19: 689-701

Lauren P. The two main histological types of gastric carcinoma: diffuse and so-callled intestinal type of carcinoma. An attempt at a histo-clinical classification. Acta Pathol Microbiol Scand. 1965; 64: 31-49.

Lee S., Kim S., Lee J., Im S. et al. Usefulness of CT volumetry for primary gastric lesions in predicting response to neoadjuvant chemotherapy in advanced gastric cancer. Abdom Imaging. 2009; 34 (4): 430-40.

Lee JH, Jeong YK, Kim DH, et al. Two-phase helical CT for detection of early gastric carcinoma: importance of the mucosal phase for analysis of the abnormal mucosal layer. J Comput Assist Tomogr. 2000; 24: 777–782.

Lee J., Lee J., Kim S. et al. Diagnostic Performance of 64-Channel Multidetector CT in the Evaluation of Gastric Cancer: Differentiation of Mucosal Cancer (T1a) from Submucosal Involvement (T1b or T2). Radiology. 2010; 255:3; 805-814.

Lee M., Choi D., Park M., Lee M.. Gastric cancer: Imaging and staging with MDCT based on the 7th AJCC Guidelines. Abdom Imaging. 2012; 37: 531-540.

Lim JS, Yun MJ, Kim MJ, et al. CT and PET in stomach cancer: preoperative staging and monitoring of response to therapy. RadioGraphics. 2006; 26: 143-156.s

Mani NB, Suri S, Gupta S, et al. Two-phase dynamic contrast-enhanced computed tomography with water-filling method for staging of gastric carcinoma. Clin Imag. 2001; 25: 38-43.

Marrelli D, Roviello F, Manzoni G, et al. Different patterns of recurrence in gastric cancer depending on Lauren´s histological type: longitudinal study. World J Surg 2002; 26: 1160-65.

Maruyama K., Sasako M., Kinoshita T. et al. "Should systematic lymph node dissection be recommended for gastric cancer? European Journal of Cancer. 1998; 10: 1480–1489.

McCulough ML, Robertson AS, Jacobs EJ, et al. A prospective study of diet and stomach cancer mortality in United States men and women. Cancer Epidemiol Biomarkers Prev. 2001; 10:1201-1205.

Meyers MA. Dynamic radiology of the abdomen, 5th Ed. New York, NY: Springer-Verlag 2000.

Merry AH, Schouten LJ, Goldbohm RA, et al. Body mass index, height and risk of adenocarcinoma of the oesophagus and gastric cardia: a prospective cohort study. Gut. 2007; 56: 1503-1511.

Monig SP, Zirbes TK, Schroder W, et al. Staging of gastric cancer: correlation of lymph node size and metastatic infiltration. Am J Roentgenol. 1999; 173: 365-367.

Moschetta M, Ianica A, Anglani A, Marzullo A et al. Preoperative staging of gastric carcinoma obtained with MDCT vessel probe reconstructions and correlations with histhological findings. Eur Radiol. 2010; 20: 138-145.

NCCN (US). NCCN Gastric Cancer Panel Members. Practice guidelines in Oncology v.2. 2009

Ng C, Husband J MacVicar A, et al. Correlation of CT with histopathological findings in patients with gastric and gastro-oesphageal carcinomas following neoadjuvant chemotherapy. Clin Radiol. 1998; 422-427.

Nitti D, Mocelin S, Marchet A et al. Recent advances in conventional and molecular prognostic factors for gastric adenocarcinoma. Surg Oncol N Am. 2008; 17: 467-83.

Pan W, Ishii H, Ebihara Y, Gobe G. Prognostic use of growth characteristics of early gastric cancer and expression patterns of apoptotic, cell proliferation, and cell adhesion proteins. J Surg Oncol. 2003; 82:104-10.

Park SR, Lee SJ, Kim CG, et al. Endoscopic ultrasound and computed tomography in restaging and predicting prognosis after neoadjuvant chemotherapy in patients with locally advanced gastric cancer. Cancer. 2008; 112: 2368-2376.

Park HS, Lee JM, Kim SH, et al. Three-Dimensional MDCT for Preoperative Local Staging of Gastric Cancer Using Gas and Water Distention Methods: a Retrospective Cohort Study. Am J Roentgenol. 2010; 195:1316–1323.

Parkin DM. International variation. Oncogene. 2004; 23: 6329-6340

Patnana M, Vikram R in New Staging System for Gastric Cancer. In D.Tan, G.Lauwers, Advances in Surgical Pathology. Gastric Cancer. Philadelphia, Lippincott, IWilliams & Wilkins, 2011. p. 266-279.

Pera M, Cameron AJ, Trastek VF, et al. Increasing incidence of adenocarcinoma of the esophagus and esophagogastric junction. Gastroenterology. 1993; 104: 510-513.

Pinheiro P, Tyczynski J, Bray F, et al. Cancer in Portugal. IARC Technical Publication No 38. Lyon, France. 2002.

Polkowski W, van Sandick J, Offerhaus G, et al. Prognostic value of Lauren classification and c-erbB-2 oncogene overexpression in adenocarcinoma of the esophagus and gastroesophagic junction. Ann Surg Oncol. 1999; 6: 290-7.

Prediction of pathologic response to neoadjuvant chemotherapy in advanced gastric cancer by MDCT: results of a prospective trial (www.rescancer.com/liver-cancer/59087.html).

49

Preto JR, Sousa JP, David L et al. A invasão venosa e a influência no prognóstico do carcinoma gástrico. Arq Port Cirurgia. 2001; 10: 80-88.

Roder JD, Bottcher K, Busch R, Wittekind C, Hermanek P, Siewert JR. Classification of regional lymph node metastasis from gastric carcinoma. German Gastric Cancer Study Group. Cancer. 1998; 82: 621-631.

Sanduleanu S, Jonkers D, D Bruine A, et al. Non-Helycobacter pylori bacterial flora during acid-suppressive therapy: differential findings in gastric juice and gastric mucosa. Alimentary Pharmacol Ther. 2001; 15: 379-388.

Sepulveda A, Goyal A. Helicobacter Pylori and Gastric Neoplasms. In: Advances in Surgical Pathology. Gastric Cancer. Philadelphia: Lippincott Williams & Wilkins, 2011. p. 22-37.

Shen KH, Wu CW, Lo SS, et al. Factors correlated with number of metastatic lymph nodes in gastric cancer. Am J Gastroenterol. 1999; 94(1):104-8.

Shimizu K, Ito K, Matsunaga N, et al. Diagnosis of Gastric Cancer with MDCT Using the Water-Filling Method and Multiplanar Reconstruction: CT–Histologic Correlation. AJR. 2005; 185:1152–1158

Shinohara T., Ohyama S., Yamaguchi T., Muto T. et al. Preoperative TNM Staging of Advanced Gastric Cancer with Multi-Detector Row Computed Tomography. JMAJ. 2005; 48 (4): 175-182.

Sobin L, Wittekind C. TNM Classification of Malignant Tumours. Wilmington, Wiley-Kiss, 2002.

Sobin L, Gospodarowisz M, Wittekind C. TNM Classification of Malignant Tumors. Hoboken: UICC-Wiley; 2009.

Takao M, Fukuda T, Iwnaga AS, et al. Gastric cancer. Evaluation of triphasic spiral CT and radiologic-pathologic correlation. J Comput Assis Tomogr. 1998; 22: 288-294.

Terres AM, Pajares JM, O'Toole D et al. H.pylori infections associated with down regulation of E-cadherin, a molecule involved in epithelial cell adesion and proliferation control. J Clin Pathol. 1998; 51:410-412.

Theuer CP, Kurosaki T, Ziogas A, et al. Asian patients with gastric carcinoma in the United States exhibit unique clinical features and superior overall and cancer specific survival rates. Cancer. 2000; 89: 1883-1892.

Uozaki H., Fukayama M.. Epstein-Barr vírus and gastric carcinoma-viral carcinogenesis through epigenic mechanisms. Int J Clin Exp Pathol. 2008; 1: 198-216.

Verdecchia A, Corazziari I, Gata G, et al. Explaining gastric cancer survival differences among european countries. Int J Cancer. 2004; 109: 737-741.

Wang W, Li Y, Sun X, Chen Y, et al. Prognosis of 980 patients with gastric cancer after surgical resection. Chinese Journal of Cancer. 2010; 11: 922-928.

Weber W, Ott K. Imaging of esophageal and gastric cancer. Semin Oncol. 2004; 31: 538-541.

Winter TC, Ager JD, Nghiem HV, et al. Upper gastrointestinal tract and abdomen: water as an orally administered contrast agent for helical CT. Radiology. 1996; 201: 365-370.

Yan C, Zhu Z, Yan M, Zhang H et al. Size of the Largest Lymph Node Visualized on Multi-detector-row Computed Tomography (MDCT) is Useful in Predicting Metastatic Lymph Node Status of Gastric Cancer. The Journal of International Medical Research. 2010; 38: 22-33.

Yang DM, Kim HC, Jin W, et al. 64 multidetector-row computed tomography for preoperative evaluation of gastric cancer: histological correlation. J Comput Assist Tomogr. 2007; 31: 98–103.

Yu J, Choi S. Choi W, Chung J et al. Value of Non visualized Primary Lesions of Gastric Cancer on Preoperative MDCT. AJR. 2007; 189: W315-W319.

.

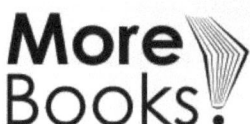
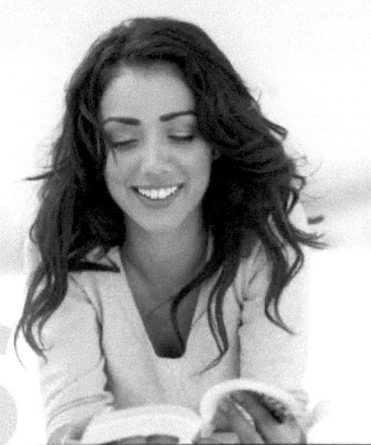

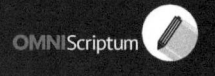

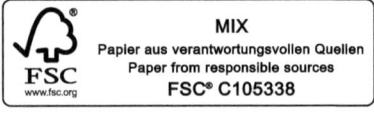
Printed by Books on Demand GmbH, Norderstedt / Germany